Breath

52 reflections for those who care for the dying

Matt Holmes

Breath:52 reflections for those who care for the dying/Matt Holmes

978-0-9827530-9-5 (paperback edition)

PSYCHOLOGY / Grief & Loss

RELIGION / Christian Ministry / Counseling & Recovery

Books may be ordered through booksellers or by contacting:

Avenida Books www.avenidabooks.com

Printed in the United States of America

Avenida Books

A|V

Contents

Breath

My kid had pneumonia. It made breath the first and last friend, the constant companion, that which quickens the dirt in the garden, a struggle to take in. It hurt him; it killed me. After the doctor's visit, my dear wife took the kid home, and I went to the pharmacy to fill the prescriptions.

I handed over the scripts and the pharmacist said it would be twenty minutes. Up until that point, the day had been nothing but fear and rushing. Appointments were set up, schedules were adjusted, a child was watched with an unblinking eye. But then, for twenty minutes, I had nothing to do but wander around the brightly-lit store. I looked at items I would never buy, and thought thoughts that weren't about life or death. It was beautiful. In that wandering, there was comfort.

When the order was finished, the pharmacist handed me the medications in a brown paper bag. Taking it in my hand, I felt its material. I heard the crunch of the paper, and I was immediately transported to my childhood, carried back to days of taking my lunch to school, its contents not albuterol and antibiotics, but peanut butter and Hostess cupcakes. For an instant, my senses brought me to a time without worries and fears. In that escape, there was comfort.

Eventually, my mind wandered to the contents of the bag. Medications, little tablets and vials of solutions—each proves the existence of illness and the pain that comes with it. Each points to the hope that the pain can be healed, that the horror can be kept at bay. In that hope, there was comfort.

My fears were largely unwarranted, the concerns of a newish dad thinking the worst. They were fears nonetheless, and that twenty minutes to wander, that brown paper bag, and those medications were comforts. Those in fear for the health and the life of their loved ones, caught up in the midst of a crisis, do not experience the worry as a momentary thing. They are awash in it, buried under the swells of terrible thoughts that are half thought and the heaviest of worries. For them, any reprieve from the pain is no small thing; it is the greatest of gifts. Today, give that gift. Allow all those who are worn out to wander from the bedside and realize that the world is larger than the sick room. Give them an instant to escape their fears. Take over the worry and they can breathe again. Give them a hope for peace and an end to suffering. In doing so, you will add some comfort to this world. That is a precious and beautiful thing.

Dirge

The overhead speaker at a hospital sings. Its song is of life and death. It can rush staff to a stopped heart when calling out its codes and it can warm hearts still beating when it plays that little nursery rhyme jingle at every birth. The speaker reminds us that within slivers of time and moments of space, lives begin and lives end.

I had a patient named John. He was the kind of guy you either loved or hated, and most hated. He was gruff and sarcastic, hilarious and often mean. Years of disease had wrapped a barbed wire around his tender heart. He struggled with illness for what seemed like ages, and for ages John drove everyone around him nuts. That is, until his grandson was born. The birth of this child did not extend John's life. No, the 52-year-old died three months later. The birth of this child did, however, allow John to die peacefully. This child, this squirming little ball of neediness and love, let John know, in unbroken flesh, that there was more to life than his death. After the birth, John's anger gave way to gratitude, cruelty to kindness. John was a man without any faith, but the birth of this child gave his last days meaning. The new life that entered this world allowed John to leave it. Life itself opened the door for John to die well.

If we leave out the great by and by and set aside notions of what comes after this world, all we are left with are the hospital speakers. The call to attend the dying and the encouragement to rejoice at new birth. For John, and perhaps for all of us, that is enough. So when our task grows hard, when it seems the only song that plays is the funeral dirge, may we remember that, somewhere, hospital speakers are playing their happy little jingle. There is always new life.

Pilgrims

This weekend my wife and I moved our kid from his crib to a big boy bed. The move was not well received. To the little guy, the bars of the crib were a comfort, something he could rely on to hold him up, to keep him safe as he slumbered, something he could depend on. Taking away his crib, while necessary, cut into his comfort, pared back his safety, and removed a sliver of his trust in this world. It was, perhaps, a first step on a road that can and often does lead to distrust and cynicism.

We are born dependent. Reliant on our caregivers for all things. It's a good thing babies don't know anything of the world they enter. It's a good thing my son was ignorant to the fact that his crib was some cheap off-brand contraption, put together in haste by his father who is about as handy as a goldfish. More than the bed, it's a good thing my son was born with no inkling of how petty I can be, how lazy and selfish. If he knew, how could he depend on me? If babies were born with a working knowledge of human weakness, childhood would be a terror of dependence without comfort, need without trust. It's a good thing children are ignorant of human frailty. Our patients are not.

It is an audacious thing we ask of them, these newly dependent people from whom freedom and strength has been stolen. We ask them—not innocent children, but seasoned adults, often adults who have faced down the horrors of a normal life and the pain of a terminal illness—to depend on us, people whom they have never met before. And what's amazing is that they do. We are welcomed as honored guests into strangers' homes. The world, with all its problems, gives us little reason to trust each other, and so there is a touch of the divine and a hint of miracle in the way our patients and families receive us. Today, may we walk in reverence as pilgrims on holy ground, as servants at the temple of the bedside, and know the honor of being entrusted with another's life and with another's death.

One in a Billion

As I understand it—and I understand it poorly—we, this, all that is and all that ever will be, is the result of imperfection. Matter is born of heat and light. All matter was born with a twin. For every drop, every ounce of matter, a drop and an ounce of antimatter was created. And since the dawn of time, there has been sibling rivalry such that matter and antimatter, when they touch, destroy each other. If the laws of physics were perfect, if the universe were symmetrical and uniform, then as quick as the universe could give birth to matter, it would mourn its death. Nothing would be left. But as it turns out, for every billion pieces of antimatter created there are a billion and one pieces of matter created. In other words, the universe is imperfect, and because of that, we exist. Each of us is one in a billion. We are the leftover, the aggregate result of the imperfect laws of physics.

Bob, the son of a patient, was imperfect. Bob was not a strong man or a smart man. By many standards his life had been a failure—a string of jobs begun and lost, a grown man living at home with his mom, few friends and little to show for himself. Bob cared for his dying mother, a task which had seemed beyond his capacities. She was older but not small; she suffered from pain and respiratory distress. She needed help with bathing and toileting. Even for those with training and strength, the task of caring for a dying person is a struggle. It seemed Bob didn't have it in him, that he was too imperfect for the task.

Nancy was an RN assigned to the case, and her vision was bigger than most. Where others would have seen only the imperfections, she saw unique strengths; where others would see only the failure, she saw the potential. Nancy saw in Bob's strength and imperfections the building blocks of a caregiver. With thought and patience, Nancy built Bob up. Bob's mother died peacefully in her home, with the best of care given by her own son. After grief and time, Bob was a different man. He had pride in the care he had given; he found meaning in the love that he showed. From that day on Bob was stronger, more confident. Through Nancy's help and the care he gave, Bob found his worth even in his imperfection. From then on Bob recognized that he is like the rest of us— one in a billion—and new life was born out of death. That, too, is a miracle.

Lake Michigan Frozen

Walking by the banks of the great inland sea, one moves away from the ramblings of lives in motion. To the right, birch trees stand white and bear the bones of the earth jutting out in endless reaching. To the left the frozen waves, the stilled motion of the breakers held perpetually in a moment, clawing against the chaos. In the suspended instant the world dances, spinning and struggling since time immortal. A husband and wife, after sixty years of marriage, begin a new ritual of holding each other's hands through the dark. They hope the grasp will keep the specter of death at bay during the night. A son throws himself on the body of his mother as life slips from her, holding her against the ceaseless pull of the inevitable. A mother returns to the hospital in the middle of the night, hoping to hold the child who only took a single breath in this world. She holds the child, feeling for what life may be left in the tiny frame. Each holding on to a moment; each clawing against the chaos.

To be human is to light and tend a candle in the ceaseless storm, to hold on to smoke, to make a moment stretch on forever. There is beauty incomprehensible in that hope and love without end. So, if in the course of today or tomorrow, you should come upon the dying or those tending to them, and should you have the time, hold their hands and remain by their sides as they claw against the chaos. In doing so, you will be privy to true humanity and a precious frozen beauty.

Mourner's Song

Some cultures demand it; others shudder to hear it. Some see it as a measure of the love lost, others as weakness. I can't recall the first time I heard it. I don't remember the dead, don't remember the family, the place, or the time of day. It must have been in the hospital, outside of some room where the specter of death had just passed. I do remember the sound, the first hearing of a song sung a million times, always heard differently and always absolutely the same—the mourner's song, the cry of someone who has lost another. The gut-wrenching call of those who have had a piece of themselves ripped from their being and from this world.

For some, it is a loud guttural response loud enough to be heard through closed doors and around corners. For others, the mourning song is something more internal, a soft cry, or perhaps relieved laughter. Whether it is screamed out for all to hear or a dirge played for an audience of one in the theater of the heart, the mourner always sings. Mourning is nothing more than a love song without a melody, the arraignment of a life lost played in one cacophonous instant. The love that has lost its object demands a body, and it takes its shape in the sounds of mourning.

Just like all of death, the mourner's song can be something ugly, something hard to hear and frightening. It can be difficult to dwell in that place with the mourner, even harder to do it day in and day out. But there is more to the mourner's cry than the ugly. Beauty can be found there. The mourner's song is built on notes of laughter as much as tears, on love as much as loss, on joy as much as pain. Any song worth singing, any tune worth playing is buried somewhere in the mourner's call, and in that way the song of the mourner can be the most beautiful of music.

The Smiling God

Can't remember when, probably at some dusty market, I picked up an icon of Jesus. It now hangs on the basement wall. In the painting, as in many icons, the Christian deity is kind-eyed and sourpussed. The serious face gazes out from the ten-by-five-inch block of wood the image was painted on. I have been told that the faithful of the Christian Orthodox church see icons as sacramental, as imbued with the spirit of God. That in some real way the painting on the wall is more than pigment and wood; that it is the very essence of Jesus. In some way, Jesus lives within the artwork.

Bowing to her children's demands, a woman who had lost her husband donated every stitch of clothing he owned within a week of his death, save one undershirt. It was tucked away in the corner of a drawer, and neither the woman nor her children noticed it during their cleanse of the home. Worn threadbare, the shirt had been a point of gentle contention between the two. She told him to throw it away, though she knew he never would. Today she sleeps in that shirt, because it is a close as she can get to lying next to him.

We do not die whole. We leave pieces of ourselves scattered through worlds we have inhabited. Slivers of our souls have leached into old t-shirts, drops of our spirit left in ripped and worn copies of our favorite books, flashes of our very lives imprinted on old photographs. But the biggest portions of ourselves we leave in those we have known. Each of you who have cared for another now harbors pieces of them inside you. We are homes for wandering souls.

When I heard this woman's story, I went home and took a look at that icon of Jesus. That stern-faced deity. I relaxed on the couch, turned on the music I like and, once comfortable, called back to mind the pieces of all those I have cared for who have left this world. They drew breath once more, if only in my mind. We sat together, and after some time I glanced up at the face on the icon and, though it was impossible and only lasted a moment, the stern-faced God seemed to smile back.

Order of Service

On Sunday, as we always do, our remnant of the faithful gathered in a worn and old church. Faded glory and ancient wisdom hung thick in the air as the musicians played the meditation before service. Just as the music quieted and the preacher drew his breath to begin, the crash of two cars colliding outside the church rang through the sacred hall.

Nobody was seriously injured in the accident, though the people involved were far from happy, and within a moment or two the police were on the scene. The church service had to continue, and so the hymns were sung accompanied by sirens as well as piano, red and blue flashes added to the flicker of candles, and the jeweled rays of sunlight passed through stained glass. The chaos of the world slipped right into the order of the service.

This could have been distracting, the holy spell of the temple broken by the profane world nudging through the door, but it wasn't. The shrill screams of the sirens made the beauty in the melodies more pronounced. The chaos of flashing lights and raised voices made the peace and order of the service appear more fragile and more precious than it had before. Order added balance to the chaos outside and chaos added body and depth to the order of the service.

A dying person is in the street, out at an accident, amongst the brokenness, the noise, and the fear. We show up among the dying with more than meds, more than strength, and more than skill. We bring expertise in the face of the unknown, calm in the face of calamity, and hope to confront despair. We walk the dying from the chaos of illness into the sanctuary of care. It is there in that place where order and chaos, life and death bleed together. It is there that miracles happen. That is the place we are blessed to do our work.

Moments and Monuments

Two men sat together as they often do, chatting. One had lost a loved one but time had passed. Raw wounds had become jagged scars, searing pain had become a dull, longing ache, an ache the man now knew would never leave him. This bereaved friend turned to the other.

"I want to thank you," he said.

"For what?" his friend replied.

"On the day she died, when I called you, you said: 'I'll be right there.' It wasn't so much that you came that mattered; it was the words. At a time of complete confusion, you gave me something to count on." The friend looked up, tears building in the rim of his eyes.

"How do you remember what I said?" he asked.

"Everything from that day is painted on my heart," the bereaved replied.

For the most part, human memory is a series of fading impressions and lingering senses, a nebulous cloud of information we draw upon to pull the scattered past back together. Most memory is fraught with discrepancies and mistakes, more a haphazardly put together reproduction of hazy events than a picture of true history. That is, except for those most painful parts of our lives. True trauma and tragedy is often marked by a perfect recall of the event, such that sentences spoken in haste can be recalled word for word years later. Talk to someone about the last breaths of their mother, spouse, child—not a second of that time will have slipped their mind, not an instant disappeared back into the ether. Though these captured instants happen at times of great strain and difficulty, they are often accented by words and deeds of astounding beauty and heroic care.

These memories are etched forever on the walls of time. These moments become monuments, canvases stained forever with the pigments of pain, comfort, and release, preserved for the ages. As we walk in these timeless lands, may we always be guided by love instead of fear, with bravery and with mercy. And in so doing, those instants will hang forever on the walls of the minds of those we have served, framed by pain and loss, but masterpieces of love and compassion nonetheless.

Working Our Way Out of the Dark

When was the last time you watched the stars burn at night? Have you stood far out past the immaterial canopy of headlights, LEDs, and 60-watt bulbs, out past the glow of the universe we have built for ourselves, and held your gaze deep into the blackened world beyond that veil? The world where eternal points still burn? I rarely get the chance to see the stars, but when I do, I watch them with the zeal of a convert. It is amazing how the longer a person looks at the sky, allowing their eyes to adjust to the infinity of space, the more the brilliant points of light slither their way through the inky void and into perception. It is as if they know you're looking. Ancient universes of indescribable power and beauty find a new home in the watching eye, given new birth in the gaze of the beholder, working their way out of the dark. In these moments, the night sky opens its gates and its treasures spill out. Truly looking at the life of another is not unlike gazing at the stars. Seeing past the clouds of ourselves and our hang-ups, looking past the dark night of our prejudice and pain, our distractions and diversions, to see the bits of beauty and light in another life poking through.

What does it mean to be the last to see the simmering beauty of another life? The last to perceive the points of light that pierce the night sky of the dying's existence?

It is there in the revealed glow of another that we meet the divine. In the light of the other, we touch that which is beyond ourselves. When we spend our time truly looking at the other, allowing the light of their life to tear the veil that separates us, and when they enter our hearts, it is there that we gaze upon the very face of God, and our task becomes our blessing.

Whispering to Ghosts

Sometimes, early in the morning, my boy will wake up calm. He usually is far from calm, screaming and rattling his crib like a caged animal. But every so often he gently pulls his consciousness from sleeping to awake. During these rare occurrences, instead of crying out, he will start the day talking to himself. At 18 months old, what he chooses to say is very interesting. Alone in his crib, he will list off a litany of the names of people he has met: Mommy, Daddy, Baba, Nana, Grandma, Grandpa, Shannon, Zack, Angela, Hope, Abbie, Max, Elmo, Ernie. Each day this list grows, and as every new person is added, the list just gets longer. So far, nobody has dropped off. Lying in bed, while part of me wishes he would just shut up so I could grab another minute or two of rest, I wonder why he does it. Why would a child, to whom the entire world is new and exciting, spend his time thinking about second cousins once removed whom he met for a couple of minutes at a barbeque?

Some people will tell you that children are born innocent. They are not, or at least my son wasn't. But he is unsullied and uninfected with the cares and desires of this world. He has yet to be confined by societal pressures or the dreams and cares of others. What he thinks about is his own, and what he chooses to think about is the people in his life. With the entire world stripped away, what matters most to the boy when he first wakes up is the people in his life. In naming them, he somehow calls them back to himself. His little bedroom is filled with memories of all his buddies.

I might not say their names, but I have found myself doing the same thing with people who have long since went to the grave, people who made an impression in my heart and stamped themselves upon my soul through the alchemy of connection. I might not call out a litany of names like the boy, but even whispers in the spirit call them back. I miss them sometimes: Mary's whit, Joe's heart, Fran's wisdom. Once in a while I think we need to bring them back, to give the dead a place before our minds once more, to breathe life into the dry bones, and from that draw the strength to continue to care for those still alive.

Pastel Beyond the Pale

On Saturday, my neighborhood had its annual Easter Egg Hunt, an event that seems to have less to do with the Christian holiday than it does with festivities in the Roman Coliseum. With the scream of the starting whistle, hundreds of children barreled toward the candy-colored plastic eggs strewn haphazardly around an open field. Elbows flew, teeth were bared, hearts broken, hopes and fingers stomped. Within thirty seconds, a torrent of tears were streaming down children's faces, a battlefield of skinned knees and stolen treasures. What did they have to show for their efforts? Sugary candy and toys that posed choking hazards to children under three, and all the kids were under three.

As Easter Egg Hunts go, it was a rousing success, and none of the pastel-clad children seemed to mind that it was a balmy 31 degrees out and overcast. If you stripped away the kids, and the toys, and the laughter, and the tears, you were left with eggs and bunnies, universal symbols of fertility and new life. The thing of it is, February sets records for its cold temperatures and March has continued this frosty trend. While the symbols spoke of new life, the world remained dead. No flowers had bloomed, grass was still brown and brittle, trees had yet to bud. This Easter Holiday confronted us with new life in a world still frozen in wintery gloom. But the kids didn't mind. They knew spring was just around the corner. We who are caring for the dying spend our working days and nights in the winter, in the times when lives become barren. Each day we encounter and care for those whose potential on this earth is all but spent. For the loving, for the caring— which each of you are—this can be brutal. The winter of death can chill us to the bone. But there is a lesson in those children bounding over frozen ground after those eggs. With winter all around, they looked to the spring just out of view, the pastel beyond the pale, the feast that will mark the end of the famine. May we who stand by the bedside always live in the hope that even as death comes, it never comes alone. Just beyond the horizon, just coming into view is its constant traveling companion. The trees will bud again, the flowers will bloom again, because wherever death goes, new life is never far behind, and there is comfort in that.

Grace in the Garden

Imagine the Last Supper: friends are gathered, food and drink are served. If everything went right, and I suppose it did, that night the upper room rang with laughter and arguments, tears and sighs, the sounds of any gathering of true friends and family. As with any good gathering, there is that point, that golden moment, when you wish it would never end. I imagine that it was at that moment, at that time, when all Jesus wanted to do was have one more glass of wine, one more laugh, one more embrace with his friends. It was at that moment that he had to go to the garden. From that point on everything would be different, and I imagine he relished those final moments in that upper room with those he loved.

Our lives are full of these final moments, most much more mundane than the Last Supper. The last drink at a party, the last day of a vacation, the last dance at a wedding. These final moments of joy are bittersweet; we savor the instant knowing that it is fleeting and hoping it or something like it will come again. There are final moments of gravity also: the last moment before a child gets on the school bus for the first time, the last class in an education, the last day of a long and meaningful career. These moments shake and form our lives, and among them is the last breath of a loved one's life.

Final moments come to us all. We may keep them at bay for as long as possible, but the night has to end, the career will see itself through; our lives cannot be lived for an eternity. When we do our jobs right, when all things work together for the benefit of those in our care, we allow others to live these last moments. We suck the marrow from final moments, see them in brilliant color, and hold those last instances forever. In that way, final moments can exist in beautiful stillness, forever.

Cracks

Two-year-olds make interesting theologians. Sometime before we moved into our home, probably in a springtime downpour, water had crept its way into the corner of my boy's bedroom and left its mark on the ceiling. A small spider web of cracks in the plaster reached out in every direction. Just a little imperfection in the paint, a crack in the plaster. Every so often he will look up at this small crack, point and say: "Jesus coming." Meaning, in two-year-old speak, that Jesus is going to, or has already entered his room through this crack in the ceiling. It's hard to know where he picked this theological tidbit up. It might have been that, somewhere along the way, as so many kids do, Hugh got Santa confused with Christ and, as many fewer kids do, the chimney confused with a crack in his ceiling. That could be, but like so many fathers, I'm sure my child is a prodigy and perhaps there is more to this observation than is immediately apparent.

While our home is older, for the most part it's in very good shape. There are a few spots of chipped paint, maybe a window or two that could use a good cleaning, or even replacing. The furnace is ancient but still works. Yet, for the most part, the house is in good shape. So what draws my son's eye to this one, small imperfection, and what makes him associate it with how he understands the divine? Why would his new mind place the transcendent in the broken? Perhaps because that is the place where goodness, where what binds all of us together and makes us better than ourselves alone, is made most apparent.

We miss the beauty in the smooth, the blessing in the unbroken, the joy in the working. When things function as they should, when traffic flows, when our bodies are strong, our work productive, there is a holiness to that harmony, but one that remains in the background, hidden from sight. It has slipped through our fingers. If we want to really see the holy, touch the sacred, we must go to the broken. We must sit in the hospital room, hold the hand of the dying, wipe the tears of the bereaved. It is there in the brokenness that the best of who we are and who we can be together becomes palpable. It is in our care for each other through the pain that the transcendent is made tangible. It is in the broken places, through the cracks in everything, Leonard Cohen wrote, that the light gets in.

The Beat of Life, The Beat of Death

I used to think of my car as an island of good tunes in a sea of pop-y nonsense. The car used to be home to Dylan & the Dead, The Stones and Talking Heads. Since my child became old enough to have an opinion, I would pay to hear Lloyd Price, and sitting through a Smokey Robinson tune would be a miracle. Nowadays Hugh cries if he can't listen to the ubiquitous songs, the Katy Perry and Taylor Swift anthems that are spread thinly across every platform from radio to TV commercials. The top forty garbage lays like a blanket over the media world, the songs we are subject to hear a hundred times a day. It's a shame but no surprise Hugh likes this stuff. Humans are designed to be drawn to the familiar.

The average heart beats between 60 and 120 beats per minute. This is the cadence of the quickening rhythm of life. I have been told that nearly every popular piece of music, every tune that resonates with large swaths of the population, matches this magic rhythm of 60 to 120 beats per minute.

Something happens to us when we hear music with this beat, a familiarity as the outside matches the inside, the harmony of the heart and human experience, the beat and the body overlap. Music that lands in that mystic 60 to 120 beats per minute is the anthem of life, and that draws us to it. A dying person's heartbeat can become erratic and chaotic, prone to sudden changes and shifts, the rhythm out of sync with that song of life. The heartbeat of the dying is dissonant, less the polished notes of a symphony and more the harsh wail of a car alarm. While the sweet spot of 60 to 120 beats is accessible to all, the heartbeat of the dying is not nearly as familiar, not nearly as pleasing. The heartbeat of the dying is not a top 40 pop song; it's Miles Davis, not Britney Spears.

We are drawn to the comfortable and fall easily into the simple and familiar, but we can find a strange beauty in the eerie, erratic rhythm at the end of a life. The song of death can carry a meaning and power all its own. Our task is to smooth out the shrill notes, to make sense of the noise. When we do our jobs right, when things go as we wish them to, our patients and families can find meaning in the end of a life. We can help people move confidently along the rhythm of death. It is our blessing and our charge to help our patients and their families find beauty in the final heartbeats and music in our last moments.

Vision

Five years ago, give or take one in either direction, I read "The Book of Disquiet" by the Portuguese philosophical novelist Pessoa. I only remember one line and I probably understand it wrong. That being said, after all these years, the phrase that still bounces around my mind is: "We are as large as our vision." Or something like that. For the past week or so I have been dealing with a sty on my eye. Besides the slight mar on the Mona Lisa-like beauty of my face, it has been among the smallest of tragedies at home or abroad.

While it is only a minor annoyance, a slight pain, the sty has decreased my field of vision, forcing me to rely heavily on my right eye, which can see about as well as a near-sighted mole. For the past week my world has become fuzzy, thin, and small. In turn, I have found myself cranky and short, irritable and small. To see small is to see with damaged vision, too tight to take it all in, too fuzzy for focus, and as our vision shrinks, we diminish along with it. Depending on our gaze, the world is either a tiny place or a cosmos endlessly complicated, interwoven, and huge. A small world is one of problems; a large world is full of potential. A small world is a world of weakness, a large world one of strength. Small worlds contain only pain; large worlds make space for relief. Small worlds only know suffering; large worlds know meaning within and beyond the suffering.

May we always see large and, in turn, may we grow to meet our vision. Grow to trust in the strength of others, to hope for wholeness beyond the brokenness, and to see our patients and their families as massive as they truly are. May we be large enough to bear another's burden just long enough to help them see their ability to carry it themselves.

Unafraid in the Land of the Dying

On Wednesdays, my kid and I go to the cemetery. If it's nice outside and we have the time, we go out among the tombs and graves, and he plays. He bounces from headstone to headstone and digs in the dirt—the boy loves the graveyard. For a child, the land of the dead holds no terror, the bodies beneath his feet no fright. When it's time to leave, the child pitches a holy fit the same as when it's time to leave Grandma's or the park. He's sad to go home because he has so much fun with the dead.

We go to the Lutheran cemetery, which sits directly north of the Jewish cemetery and south of the Bohemian graveyard, just east of First Ave. These cemeteries are located here because this is the spot where the train line used to end nearly a century ago. It was the last stop for Chicago public transportation. In other words, the cemeteries were formed as far from the city and the living as possible without being out of reach. You can judge a society by how they treat their animals and their dead. We aren't bad to our pets, but we want as little to do with our dead as possible. We like them just on the edge of our vision, the land of the dead a blurry haze deep in our periphery. Often the same goes for the dying, tucked away in hospitals or facilities removed from the land of the living even before they draw their last breath.

Like the cemeteries, the dying are pushed just to the limits of our reach. You who care for the dying serve as a foil to this. Part of your duty is to open the gates to the land of the dead and dying and let a little life in. It is through your kindness, your bravery, and your love that people can become a little more like my child, who walks unafraid in the land of the dying. Then they, like my son, can find a measure of comfort among the tombs. In helping others come to the dying, in helping them to stand by the bedside, we allow those leaving this world to finish their days well and loved, surrounded by those they care for in the land of the living.

Mother's Day

I don't know what it is like to be a mother. I can't image carrying new life in my guts, or the process of pushing that life out into the world, but I do know the commitment it takes just to keep a child alive. They say that human gestation is nine months in the womb and two to three years outside of it, longer than any other creature walking God's green earth. We are born broken; we are born weak, unable to sustain our own existence for more than a matter of hours. It's only through the strength of our mothers that we survive. To be a mother is to continue to care for your child. To care for them when they are good and cute, sweet and clean, and to care for them when they are vicious and mean, selfish and dirty. To be a mother is care for a child when you would rather not, when you cannot, when it hurts. To be a mother is to care for a child because, if you don't, if the child is left to their own devices, that child will not live. Just to see a child live until adulthood is a task beyond comprehension, motivated by a thick, rich love beyond explanation or end dates.

Motherhood is to give all of yourself so that the other may live. By virtue of the simple fact that they are alive, we can be sure that those who have entered our care, at least for a time, have been on the receiving end of this love. Our patient's very life proves that, for a moment, they were at the center of another's universe. They were the complete focus and total recipient of another's love and care. May each of us take a lesson from the billions of sainted mothers who have lived and loved in this world. May those in our charge find a home at the center of our worlds, if only for a moment. May they be the focus of our care as if their very lives depended on it, because in many ways they do. May we be as mothers to those we serve, giving deeply of ourselves so that the other may know life and once again feel maternal love.

A Thirtieth of a Second

Mary looked at a picture of herself at a party, a candid shot with her at the center. It was taken a month after her husband, her love, her partner, her friend, had died. The image was of a graduation party for a nephew of hers. In the picture, people were smiling, dancing, drinking, eating, living. Mary was smiling, too, but a year later, as she examined the photo, in a thirtieth of second, a sliver of time—Mary saw in that moment a difference between herself and the other partygoers; something separated them.

From her husband's diagnosis until sometime after his death, Mary had lived in a fog. Her mind, dulled by fear and then grief, was like a thick haze that stood as a veil between her and the world. In the image, she was among her friends and family, but separate from them, in this world, but touching nothing. Even as she could see this about herself in the picture, she noticed a difference in the eyes of those around her. A few sets of eyes were planted squarely on Mary; friends and family looking on, their gazes thick with a sympathy that bordered on sorrow. They saw her as a ragged thing, once beautiful, now forever scarred and broken. Most just looked away, as if to cast one's vision on someone who so recently had been acquainted with death would be to invite the shadow into their own lives.

We can see with different eyes—we who know the unceasing and pervasive presence of death and dying in the world, we for whom the final breath is not exotic, but common. We can see those losing and those who have lost with eyes of care, of empathy and not sympathy, of love and not fear. We can see them not as suffering but as people who suffer, not as the grieving but as people living with grief. We can cast a gaze that sees the person before the pain, the life before the loss, and perhaps in the reflection of our eyes, those who loved and lost can find a glimmer of hope for the future.

Thirst

Does a patient or their family every offer you a bottle of water, or a cup of coffee when you show up for a visit? Do you ever think about why? What does someone who can't be sure of their next breath care if you're a little parched or in need of a shot of caffeine? Shouldn't they worry about their own issues before they get involved with yours? Maybe, maybe not.

Questions like these fail to take into account the essential fact that, as people, we are more than our basic needs. That caring for something, be it a person, or a dog, or a garden, a work of art, or anything else—is at the center of our humanity. I visited a bereaved man last week, a man who since the loss of his wife has struggled to meet even his own basic needs. I went to care for him, but before I could offer active listening or talk about coping mechanisms, he offered me something to drink. This man, who had struggled for weeks to get out of bed, had made a special trip to the store just to pick a drink up to have something to offer. This small act was a great kindness, a good deed. Where are such acts of kindness created? What led this man and the thousands of others before and after him to reach out, even when they were in need of a hand themselves? These acts of care come from the same place that pushes people to throw baby showers for coworkers and to spend their days and their nights caring for the dying. What brings about these good works, these acts of care, is born in the very deepest part of us: the soul of our souls, our secret heart.

This is the place where the divine resides in each of us and where love and care are breathed into existence. The very center of our being is the source of love for the other. The greatest thing we can do for another is to recognize that secret heart, that temple to the holy in each of us—to know the infinite love that has chosen to make a home in our soul, and allow them to see that love in each of us.

Newborn

I have to rush to the keyboard before it fades away. Type furiously before the last traces drift off into the ether and travel to a new place, or settles into another home. Only a hint remains, still clinging to the fibers of a dirty shirt—a few strands of hair. The scent of birth has flooded my world as it has flooded all others, but the tide will inevitably go out again.

There is a smell to birth, not the new baby smell of Hallmark cards and nostalgic parents' tears, but something more visceral, more complicated, more profound. The first time each of our virgin lungs sucked in the air with all the sweet and poison scents it is laced with, we smelled it. At the birth of our children it once again fills our lungs. It is the first incense filling the temple. The scent of birth carries to the divine throne room visceral prayers of hope and a dirge for pain yet unfelt; beautiful and terrible all at once.

The smell of new birth is pain. A mother's sweat and labor, a father's worry, an infant's fear. It is pain yet unfelt, failure and loss, heartaches and illness, and eventually death. Inevitable. It is joy unbound, all things new, pure potential. An olfactory unending, perfectly recognizable and infinitely strange.

It is the aroma of a full manger and an empty tomb, different from all other scents and yet containing the cosmos. In the scent of life, pain, and hurt, love and joy twist together and rise into the atmosphere. It is all things, but different from each. On final examination, it is perhaps the only unequivocally good thing in the world. I may never smell the scent of birth again, and if I don't, well I have had enough, and that is fine. Thank you God, and love, that I smelled it today.

Whale Fall

When a whale dies, after the great beast's mammoth frame has slipped beneath the waves and settled to the ocean floor, from its lifeless frame a universe of organisms are born and nurtured. The decaying form gifts new life to scores of creatures, to wandering scavengers, to the ocean floor on which it lands. Dozens of species have been discovered which exist only on these whale falls settled on the bottom of the world, some living off of one body for ninety years. Something as distasteful as the decaying corpse of a whale means life to thousands of God's creatures. Sometimes, what seems worthless can be the greatest blessing. It was a pill; a collection of various chemicals crushed up and stirred together.

The component parts of the pill have little value on their own, elements and compounds found all around us in the air and the soil, plastic and paper. But together in the correct amounts and forms they can ease pain, cure illness, save lives. Just a little pill made from the ordinary things of our world can change a life for the better. Sometimes, what seems the tiniest of things can be the greatest blessing. What will matter, what will change the way things are does not come with a sign.

What will touch a life, what will build up the broken, heal the wounds, can be hard to see before its work is done. Tonight the care we give may simply be our duty, or it may be hope. The kind word we offer may just be conversation, or it could make all the difference. We cannot know ahead of time what will matter and what will simply pass away, but what we can do is offer what we have and who we are. At times it may not feel like much in the face of death and illness, but it can matter. If the decaying corpse of a whale can provide life for millions of organisms for a century, if a few chemicals crushed up and encapsulated together can ease pain, surely we have something to offer. Sometimes what seems so humble, so inadequate, can be the greatest blessing.

In Our Place

There is a couple who live across the street from me, a husband and wife. He's 91; she's 90. She's a talker; he hardly says a word. They're Polish immigrants who fled horrors at home to make a home in this country. A few weeks ago, as my dear wife was waddling her way down the street and through the end of her third trimester carrying our daughter, the wife in the couple across the way called out in her thick Polish accent:

"When is the baby due?"

"Any time now," my wife replied. Quietly, almost under his breath, the husband who was sitting next to his wife on the porch leaned in and said:

"Our replacement."

Meaning, I believe, that as his time on this earth draws to an end, our little girl will fill the spot he had occupied. She will take up the vacant space left behind when he sheds his mortal coil. Most people will never see their life in this vein; most people will never understand their death as making space for new life, the end of their possibility opening up avenues for others. Most people will never think about the gift and blessing it is for one life to give way to the other, but it is a gift and blessing nonetheless. The beautiful thing about our world, its endless hope, is that the hole left behind after a death will be filled again, that every death makes way for new and expansive life. In helping people die, in easing the pain of their transition and allowing their final moments to be peaceful, we honor that last noble act. We provide blessing for the final selflessness; we allow one world to fade away gently as new universes burst into existence.

Nothing to Offer

If you have ever had a newborn, you know what I am about to say is true, but you're probably smart enough to have kept it to yourself. Newborn babies are good for nothing. They demand and demand and offer nothing in return. They give no sweet smiles, they are months from a real hug, a year or so from saying "I love you." It seems a mistake of evolution that at the point when a human can offer the least in return is the very moment when they demand the most. Yet humans keep having babies, and by and large, those babies are cared for. Why?

I think it's because we don't actually care for the babies, but for the potential they harbor—the worlds they will inhabit and create, the love they will show, the things they will produce, the things they will change and the things that will change them. To care for a baby is to honor the filled manger and the potential life it represents. The dying, too, are needy with nothing to offer.

Life follows its circuit and the end resembles the beginning. By and large the dying are cared for also, but why? In caring for the dying we do not honor life in its potential, but the potential that has been realized. We honor the love that has been given, the plans fulfilled, the material created, the experiences that have been shared. In caring for the dying we show that that life and the one who lived it has mattered, that their days have had value. Even if we don't know the entire story of a life, we have faith that that life is worth serving, and that faith is a virtue. To care for the dying, to care for those who have created the worlds in which we have been blessed to live.

Small Resurrections

I, like all of you, am often asked if this work makes me sad. Does spending day after day steeped in that facet of life so hidden in plain sight, so pervasive and yet taboo as death, wear upon a soul? My answer is, for the most part, "no." I, like all of you, have found a way to live with and to understand death so that watching it, living in its wake, is no longer much of a struggle. But when I answer "no," like any conclusive statement, I am only telling a half-truth.

Leaving out kids and tragedy, the thing that tears me up about this job is often the good stuff, the things we would call "wins." The mock wedding that takes place months before the real thing so grandma can watch her first grandchild tie the knot, the last trip to the casino, the few bites of a treasured recipe, a few pulls of a final smoke or tugs off a bottle of beer—these last events that few and lucky people choose to experience before their time on this earth ends. These things have always made me sad. To me they seem too small to cap lives, too forced to be authentic, too pathetic to mark the end of a person's time on this earth, oh, but do I know.

There seems to be more going on in these last hurrahs than meets the eye. They seem to be less about the experience itself and more about the life that has been lived. Less about the taste of the particular meal and more about all the dinners shared with loved ones over the years. Less about a few hours pouring coins into a shiny box and more about the jackpots won, the adventures lived. These last experiences are slivers of beauty past, small resurrections before the death. These last things breathe a bit of life back into dying bones and ensure that nothing is wasted. They truly become occasions for great joy.

Prayer Cards

The other day I was cleaning out my office. In the midst of shredding documents and tossing detritus, I came upon a stack of funeral prayer cards. Those laminated three-by-five inch pieces of paper often included a sweet picture of the deceased on it—the date of birth and death, funeral information and the 23rd Psalm, the Lord's Prayer, or some quasi-religious, but always heartfelt poem. I couldn't bring myself to toss them.

They say if left to fend for itself, after about one millennia, all the material we humans have made will either have broken up and returned to the earth or be so worn as to be unrecognizable. Libraries will be nothing but heaps of petrified wood, buildings fallow fields, cities forest and plains. The only material which will not give into time and the elements, the only stuff of our existence which will survive to near infinitude, is plastic. There, thousands of years from now, once we are all dead and gone, in a buried layer of existence interspersed between soda bottles and Barbie dolls, will be those laminated prayer cards, eternally reminding the universe of the individuals who have faded out of existence. Our lives, as with the world, hold on to very little.

The people we encounter tend to be brushed out of our memories by time and distance, their memories worn down to nothing. But there are those people we choose to let in, those people we affect and allow to affect us in deep, authentic, and profound ways. They are stamped on our hearts, laminated into our souls. When our lives are through, when our times have come, they will be the last to go: enduring pieces of the other that have made a home in us, and in turn have given us meaning. Meeting and caring for these people is the true blessing of our task—and a great gift of this work.

Elongated

It starts with a race I always win. Once I have finally caught him, I am subject to a barrage of punches and kicks, screams and bites usually not seen outside of Black Friday shopping and The Jerry Springer Show. Then I wrestle the boy down on the changing table and get him clean and dry. By then he has usually calmed down and will innocently ask if "Daddy will lay down with me," so I lay in the bed with the child while he ever so slowly drinks his sippy cup of milk. After he finishes, I leave my son alone for his nap. This usually happens three times a day.

It is a slow, frustrating, inconvenient process to get the boy to sleep. The fact of the matter is it's a huge hassle, and the fact of the matter is I'm gonna miss it like crazy when these days are gone. The time we spend together with those we love, be it struggling or laughing, is nothing short of sacred, no matter how difficult it is.

When we meet people at the end of their ropes, battered and bruised by the demands of holding another's life in the palm of their hands, we are meeting them on holy ground. We step into their sacred time. Though caring for another in their final days is trying, those final days are a time distilled, moments elongated and stretched. The final instants with a loved one can be as brief as a blink of the eye and as long as a lifetime. May we honor this sacred space and help the other to occupy it fully, because the fact of the matter is that those final moments are a huge hassle, and the truth of the matter is that our families are gonna miss them like crazy when they are gone.

Between the Dark and the Flame

On the weekends, if it is nice outside, I like to have a fire after dark. No great shakes, just a few sticks, a couple logs wreathed in flames in my tiny fire pit. It usually doesn't take long to get the fire going, and once the wood is caught and burning on its own I'll plop down in my lawn chair, kick my feet up on an overturned five gallon bucket like the class act I am, grab a cold beverage and take a sip. It never fails that before I can take a second pull, the flames have either begun to die out or grow too hot. The wind has turned, kicking a column of smoke in my eyes, or else the logs need to be shifted before those ever-fragile flames can burn out.

The entire night will go this way. I'll get the fire just how I like it, have enough time to sit back and enjoy the warmth for a moment, and then something changes and I need to move again. A constant recalibration, a dancing with the chaotic flames, all of which is done just to maintain that sweet spot, that elusive place where the burning flames and the cold night meet to produce comfort and warmth.

Sometimes I think that is what we do; we help people find the sweet spot around the deathbed. The place where a family member can show their care and love for the dying, but with enough help and support that they don't get burned by the pain. We help the dying find where they can be with the ones they love, the place they can occupy at the end of their life so that they don't get left out in the cold. It is a moving target ebbing and flowing with the fluidity of love and memory. The art of our craft is to help find that spot between the dark and the flame, where families and patients can live and move, love and die in the warmth and comfort of each other's care.

The Temple and the Wailing Wall

My ten-week-old can smile and that's about it. She can't walk or dance or sing. She has yet to eat solid food or mow the lawn. She hasn't worked a day in her life so, of course, no paychecks. She can only smile, but what's a smile, anyway?

When you consider the universe, the vast empty space of it all, punctuated only here and there by the light of stars, a few mounds of matter—when you think about how, even in those small pockets of something instead of nothing, even there life has only been seen on this planet, and most of that life is unmoving and unthinking outside of pure instinct—a smile may be more than it would first appear. When you consider it in the grand scheme of it all, a smile, a sign of happiness, an outward representation of an inward state given for its own sake, is truly a rare and remarkable thing. While compared to an active adult, my child's abilities in the world are greatly limited. When held up next to all else that exists, her simple smile becomes nothing short of astounding.

Our patients also are often limited. What abilities they had, what powers were at their disposal, have been ripped away by illness and time. Who they were: diminished; what they could do: stolen, but that doesn't mean they don't have value, and that doesn't mean they aren't remarkable. From the mumbled prayer of the comatose to the song of the demented, even taking that last breath, that last filling of the lungs with the spirit is an act of such rare beauty as to be almost unheard of in this universe. May we honor all life for what it is: the home for the divine, and pay homage to every death as a Wailing Wall, the remnant, the echo of where the holy had dwelt within the profane.

A Gift in the Storm

Last Thursday morning I attended a funeral, and last Wednesday evening I sat with a family in the hospital as they came to see the body of a young man before it was taken into the coroner's care. Ostensibly, these two events were nearly the same. In each case loved ones came from all around to be together and to be in the presence of the material left behind after the death of their loved one. In each case they cried, they laughed, they prayed, and they mourned, and yet, these two events could not have been more different.

A funeral is order tinged with the chaotic. It follows a course, moves in channels well worn and cut by the endless streams of black-clad mourners who have darkened church doors and funeral parlor lounges. The words and prayers have a cadence recognized by all, and in that routine the magic of familiarity and order gives scaffolding on which to hang powerful emotions. The hospital room, the dying chamber, is often devoid of these predictable comforts. In those moments just after a death, where the flesh still contains a dim ember of the life that had burned out, where the blood is still damp and the bed is the one on which the act of dying has taken place, those comforts of the ordinary are no comforts at all.

The hospital room is all chaos; order simply lingers on the margins, providing only borders. When we are there in those chaotic times, in those final moments of a life and those first moments of death, we can be an anchor. Something for the families and loved ones to hold fast to as the world tosses and turns wildly around them. We are the skilled, the trained, and the experienced. We are those whose very presence tell the bereaved that they are not alone, that they stand in the company of millions who have known that same pain, and that they, like all those before them, will find a new life on the other side of chaos. In that way, your very presence is a gift and a comfort. The greatest of honors, humbling and powerful.

The Key to the Gates of Heaven

Have you ever been thirsty on an airplane? It's the worst. Maybe you had to run to the gate to make the flight just in time, perhaps you had one too many cocktails in the airport lounge, or maybe the dry air and cabin pressure had drained you of your vital fluid. For whatever reason, you find yourself parched at 35,000 feet crammed into a little seat, unable to do anything to help yourself. Tell me when that flight attendant finally hands you that little cup with a shot of water and one deformed cube of ice, if you're lucky, floating in it. Tell me when that water comes that you don't savor every drop and feel some profound sense of gratitude toward the flight attendant who brought it to you.

Same goes if you're hungry. Somehow that little bag of Gardetto's or five honey-roasted peanuts turns into a feast. Each morsel has to be chewed slowly with thought and reverence for the flavor and the sustenance they provide. The point is to say that, when you find yourself in a place where you have no power to do for yourself, when you must rely on others to meet your needs, to provide for you, the simplest things can gain great importance and the ordinary can become the extraordinary.

How much more for our patients? For those not confined by rivets and steel, but by their own flesh and bone? How much more for those whose most basic of powers have evaporated from their being? Those for whom a walk down the hall might as well be a marathon, and a mouth full of food can be a death sentence? For them water is not just water, it is liquid life; a bath is not just a bath, it is a touch of dignity they used to take for granted; relief from pain is not just relief, it is the freedom to find some of the existence which has been taken from them. These are gifts given and blessings bestowed. In everything that you do, every last act of kindness, every gentle touch is no small thing. It is relief born into this world and love given form. Even a sip of water given to one in need is no less than a key to the gates of heaven.

Ash Wednesday

My infant son received his ashes for the first time today. As the pastor's hand left its dark void on his forehead in the shape of a cross, my heart broke.

You can say what you will about religious rituals, but the event that takes place in and out of Churches around the world on Ash Wednesday is nothing if not true. In the imposition of ashes words are said that apply to all people, but words which are normally shied away from. "Remember that you are dust, and to dust you shall return." I, as much as most, am aware of the truth of this statement, and yet, when these words were applied to my toddler, I could not help but think, "not him." Not that child, not a child, not one whose life is still potential, not one whose form has yet to be broken and worn by age and illness. I may be dust and dust may be where I will find my end. Sure, the guy next to me is dust, Tom down the block and Sue around the corner—they are all dust, but not the child. Even in that same thought my mind turned to the year before, when it was my hand placing the ashes.

Placing ashes on foreheads that were undeniably dust. Hospice patients in hospitals, nursing homes, or set up in hospital beds looking out their living room windows. Bodies whose earthiness was their main attribute, forms slowly wasting away, returning to the elements from which they came. These patients were dust and their return to dust was near. That dust is holy.

Mary was dust, her body riddled by cancer, unable to leave her bed for the last six months of her life, and yet this dust had raised three children as a widow, children who went on to be good and thoughtful people. If Mary was dust, then dust is a stronger thing than we give it credit for. Joe was dust, his body broken and twisted from birth, and yet his sense of humor never left him his entire life, and will live on in his grandson, whom he loved fiercely. If Joe was dust, then dust is a hardier thing than we give it credit for. Sue was dust, her body marked and torn from the scars of a life of mental illness and the abuse that comes with it, and yet Sue had a kind word and a smile for anyone who entered her room. If Sue was dust, then dust is more loving than we could ever know. Time and time again we humans, we collections of dirt and dust, are able to do the most amazing and the most stunningly simple of things. So yes, in the end the boy is dust, our patients are dust, I am dust, and you are dust. And thank God for that.

After

Resurrection

Should you attend a liturgical church, you may notice something on a certain Sunday. During the Gospel reading, the lector will tell the well-worn story of doubting Thomas. While the readings of the church year cycle and change, a few readings remain fixed in place, read every year on the same day. Thomas' story is one of those readings. In it the Saint doubts that the man who stands before him is Jesus raised from the dead, and the proof he requires is to see and touch the wounds that the cross has left on the dead and raised body. Upon seeing these wounds, for the first time in the Bible story, Thomas calls out: "My Lord and my God."

In a religion that over a third of the world follows, the divine is known as the God in weakness. God is not found in the halls of power, nor on a throne in Rome, in the twisting spires of the Kremlin, nor in the elongated circle in Washington. God is found broken and scarred, wounded and bruised. God dwells in a small room of no consequence to the world. There are great and meaningful theological implications to this, but what matters to us is that room. That small and inconsequential room, that room where the nervous and lost are gathered. A room where the sick and the dying take the center; that is a room we all know well.

It is in these rooms, be they homes or hospitals, at times of great fear and worry, times when the very scent and feel of death and loss hangs among the gathered. It is there that the divine can be best seen and where our holy work is done. In the love of the family who has left their lives to be with the dying, the divine's love is made known. In the struggle of the dying to hold on to be with the ones they have loved just one more time, the strength of the divine is made known. In the tender mercy of the worker who attends lovingly to the needs of the dying, the compassion of the divine is made known. You are those that tread this holy ground; you are those whose hands are used for that divine work. May the labor and love that you give on this holy ground be always blessed.

Perfection

I was in a wedding not too long ago. It was a beautiful affair. The bride and groom had paid attention to every detail: the music was elegant yet fun, the food gourmet yet approachable and delicious, the décor tasteful and refined.

If you had asked the happy couple before the service how they would want their wedding described, they might have said elegant, classy, fun or warm. But if they answered honestly, they would have said, "Perfect." Like nearly all brides and grooms, they wanted every note of music played to be beautiful, every word of the sermon to be powerful, every picture to be stunning. That's what they wanted. Thank God we don't always get what we want.

The father of the bride gave his daughter away, and as he attempted to step over the bride's ridiculously long train, he kicked over one of the votive candles. The fire was put out quickly, but the dreams of perfection went up in smoke. The room erupted in laughter. As the groom turned around, everyone in the bridal party heard him mutter "Thank you," under his breath. The father of the bride's clumsy mistake was the first wedding present given that day. The spell was broken and the people relaxed. Any elegance lost was replaced with authenticity, perfection traded for pleasure, great expectations with good times.

So often we desire a perfect life, and even more a perfect death. We want our final minutes to be lived out like in the movies. With a last dignified breath we will drift off into the dark surrounded by the ones we love, peacefully and painlessly, having said everything without a single regret. Spend a little time with death and you know better. We know that dying is hardly beautiful, that it is rarely attractive, but that it can be meaningful. Our job is not to make death perfect, but to make it authentic to the dying. To let people be themselves until their last breaths. We help them to love what they love, to feel what they feel, and to live as they live until the last moment of their lives. We can't make death perfect. It's not supposed to be. But you can help it be peaceful, and you can point to its meaning. In doing so, you can give a true final gift.

Quiet Love

Have you ever gone to a two-year-old's birthday party? Have you been to one of your niece's dance recitals? Have you ever sweat through a graduation ceremony with someone else wearing the cap and gown? Have you cared for the physical needs of a dying parent? Balled your eyes out at a funeral when all you wanted to do was stay home? Spent a night sitting upright with worry or tossing and turning, trying to hide from the sorrow that won't let you sleep?

Why do we do these things? With such precious little time in this world, why do we spend one moment doing something that doesn't make us happy? Why do we sign on to things that aren't comfortable or fun?

It might have something to do with the fact that comfort can't compete with connection. Fleeting enjoyment takes a back seat to family and friends. The deep, lasting joys of relationships with others far exceeds passing pleasures. We sit through the recital, we sweat in the gym, we hold the hand of the dying because that's why we are here. That's what makes us people. Beyond the boredom of watching that two-year-old try and fail to blow out the candles is love in quiet action. Love is being there even when it isn't fun, even when it isn't pretty, even when it hurts, because being there matters more than the pain.

It is our sacred task and our solemn joy to allow love to quietly act at the end of our lives. It is our task to create the conditions for care in a way that helps people be people up until the moment of death and beyond.

Insignificant Miracles

There are a few things common among us first-time parents. Chief among them is the ubiquitous belief among all parents that their kid is the smartest, most advanced, kindest and most astounding child ever to exist. This belief of other parents is ridiculous because obviously only my child is the smartest, most advanced, kindest, and most astounding child ever to exist. Just like the rest of them. I think it is more than simple pride that leads parents to conclude that their child is uniquely gifted beyond all others. I think it comes from watching a life grow up close. It is breathtaking to watch a little mind grasp a new concept, fumbling paws master holding a fork, fat unwieldy tongues wrestling out a new word. Nearly every person accomplishes each of these acts of brilliance. Still, watching children master these most ordinary of activities transforms them into nothing less than miracles.

To watch a life grow, change, and burn is to watch an insignificant miracle. The repeated cycle of birth, growth, and death can melt hearts and leave even the divine speechless, save for gentle tears.

Dying adults are past the age of miracles, or so it would seem. Their skills have been mastered, their magic made mundane. It is up to us to find the miracles still alive in the dying, no matter how insignificant, to see them as their parents had so many years before. Then to take that beauty and hold it up before the dying once again, for the last time. To let them see how brightly their ordinary lives have burned. Today may our hands and our hearts be tools to reflect the insignificant miracles of the dying.

Truth and Death

Have you ever seen someone die? Well, of course you have. Have you ever held a person's hand as the quickening slipped through his or her lips? Yes. Have you ever washed a dead body, honoring who that person was and what that body did by gently cleaning and preparing it? Often. Have you hung around when death came calling? I guess you have. It's your job. You know death, you know its weight and its smell, its silent thunder, its opaque invisibility. You are among those who know death while most remain unacquainted. Everyone knows someone who has died, but few know death.

Death remains something we shy away from, and why not? Our world treasures two things above all else: our comfortable falsehoods and the notion of power. We will, and have, fought and killed to protect these things; the problem is, while we love the falsehood, death speaks nothing but the truth. Life is not always beautiful. Most of what we hold dear, most of the ideas and ideologies that motivate us, do not matter at all in the end. And like it or not we, each and every one of us, will die. And therein lies the proof that, while we wish to believe we are in power and that this world has bowed to our control, death reminds us incontrovertibly that we, in fact, are not in control. No wonder most find death distasteful and pretend it is only some exotic condition easily kept at bay through multivitamins and regular checkups.

I imagine you all get the same questions I am often posed with: "How do you do it? How do you remain by the deathbed? How do you linger in the dying room?" For those who see death as an affront to the half-truths and false power they cling to, choosing to dwell among the dying is insane at best and foul at worst. But we know there is more to death. There are good and powerful things in the dying room, things that cannot be found anywhere else. In a world where lies are the norm, the truth of the deathbed is itself a hidden treasure. In a world obsessed with dominance and control over all things, there can be found a freedom in the dying's fragility and liberation in the dying's limitations. The dying allow themselves to become part of the world instead of rulers over it. So when people ask me what allows me to linger in the presence of the dying, what draws me to deathbeds, I tell them: "Near the dying is the last place left in this world free of all the bullshit." Perhaps we should all stop by once in a while.

Wisdom

They say that wisdom can be found in the most unexpected of places, that she does not only dwell in dusty old books, well-worn sayings, and that smoky myth of common sense. Perhaps the start of knowing wisdom is to see that there is no place where she is not.

Elisabeth was 70. She lived in a single room above an abandoned furniture store in the part of town the good folks avoid after dark. It was a home for women in recovery—recovery from drugs and alcohol, recovery from abuse and violence, recovery from lives misspent and lives mistreated. When I met Elisabeth, cancer had already torn its way through her body. Her blood was tainted by AIDS, her liver blackened by cirrhosis, and her lungs scarred by COPD. The life she had led was killing her, and Elisabeth knew it. She faced that death heroically, beautifully, with her eyes wide open. In the end, she welcomed the pale specter as an old friend.

Elisabeth did what she could to mitigate the pain. She did not hesitate to take her meds or call the nurse for help. She did so not out of fear, but out of a desire to get the distractions of pain and discomfort behind her so that she could get on with the business of living truly and dying well. She reconnected with a brother she had not spoken with in years. She told those she loved about that love. She made good on her debts and forgave her debtors. She set up her own cremation and memorial services. Elisabeth offered final words of wisdom to those around her. She blessed her friends by letting them care for her. And when death arrived, Elisabeth was able to say something few can say, and even fewer can mean: "I have nothing left to do in this life but to die."

Elisabeth was a 70-year-old dying drug addict with AIDS, and she had more to teach me about death and life than any book, class, or sermon ever could. In our patients are endless stores of wisdom. Fonts overflowing with lessons learned through struggle and fires of life passed through. Many were burned by life's flames along the way, and many were left more beautiful for it. May we always be open to the wisdom and courage we are confronted with in deathbed after deathbed. Perhaps a piece, just a touch of who the wise, dying patients were will become a part of us.

Fireworks

The fourth of July has come and gone again, and this year, as in every year before, millions of people like me celebrated deep love for this land by blowing up a small piece of it. It is strange that of all ways to celebrate, fireworks are how we as Americans choose to mark the birth of the nation. Historically, Americans have thought of themselves as practical people, down to earth and not given to flights of fancy. We are people who build things to last and take care of what we have, people who look toward the future—and yet, on the most American of holidays we celebrate with something as frivolous and temporary as fireworks.

Fireworks are beauty born only to die. Fire and light are held for only an instant against the endless darkness of a summer night. By their very design, fireworks exist only for a moment and then fade into the black, leaving the night unchanged and unscarred by their presence. They make no lasting impact; they serve no greater purpose than a moment of pleasure and awe for the observer. Perhaps it is not simply the fire and light that makes fireworks beautiful, but the fact that they draw us out of the river of time and set us firmly on the shore of that moment. Fireworks arrest our mind and our gaze in a moment of beauty and hold us, a people so obsessed with tomorrow and with what is permanent, in an awe-inspiring instant.

Life itself is a firework. A life is a shining instant on the endless dark sky of time. Life is an explosion of fire and light that is beautiful and meaningful but seen only once and lost forever to time, which remains unchanged and unscarred. The beauty of this moment of life can often be lost. Our time with the dying is not meant to last, but to fade into the darkness of time. It is our task to find meaning in the moments. To observe the fire and light of a life ending and see value there. May we who spend our days with those that spend their last always sit in hushed awe at life now fading into that blackness, and may we live in reverence to the last sparks of fire and the light that burns in the other.

Tragedy

Tragedy is a stretchy phenomenon. It can strike with pinpoint accuracy, tearing apart one life while leaving the ones around it untouched and unscathed, or it can sprawl out, expanding its edges to catch an entire family or community. Every so often, tragedy can fall across entire nations, or perhaps the world, covering all things as a cloud or a funeral pall. Maybe it's just me, but it seems that lately tragedy has been stretching itself thin, touching all of us where we live and beyond. It has rained down upon our world at home and abroad, poured out over city streets, leaked into our work, and found the cracks in our homes.

At times tragedy can seem so close that its breath warms our necks. Children losing parents, strange illnesses affecting younger people—all death carries with it tragedy, but the tragedy of potential unrealized and of childhood cut short has a sting all its own. In times like these, our task becomes more difficult. Heavier yokes, greater struggles. In times like these, an already heavy burden can seem crushing.

The weight of tragedy will lighten. In the blink of an eye it will move on; the heavy storm will pass, bringing its burden to others, and we will be left to face the more measured loss we have grown accustomed to. In the meantime, let those around us help with the burden, lighten the load. May the very difficulties we face bind to one another in mutual care. In that way, the tragedy does not remain as simply negative, but it is transformed, transfigured into the fuel by which strength and unity grow. The burden becomes the blessing, and the strain becomes our strength.

Fat Tuesday

The 'fat' in Fat Tuesday does not refer to how you feel after an evening of drinking or eating. It has nothing to do with masks, parades, New Orleans, Rio, beads, booze or anything else commonly associated with the Mardi Gras festivities. The 'fat' in Fat Tuesday refers simply to that family of organic compounds we call fats.

In those days before refrigeration, when salt and cellars where the main means of preserving food through the long winter months, if you had not eaten your fatty foods by this point in the year, they would rot. So there was a feast before the famine. The last of the rich fatty foods were consumed, followed by a time of discipline and sacrifices needed to get through the winter alive. Fat Tuesday marks the end of abundance and the start of scarcity, the end of being full and the beginning of starvation, the movement from easy life to the very real possibility of approaching death.

When looked at in this way, it seems that Mardi Gras should be a somber event. A time when we slowly savor all that remains in thoughtful contemplation of the hard times ahead. A funeral dirge, a warning of approaching pain, but of course it isn't. Today is a day of reckless abandon, a day to set aside the worries of tomorrow and live in the moment. As the preacher says, "let us eat, drink, and be merry, for tomorrow we die."

It is precisely on the precipice of death that life is seen for the precious and fragile commodity it is. In these moments, on the edge of darkness, the light of life burns brightest. We guide people through these moments. Our best and only true response to approaching death is to celebrate the life that remains with reckless abandon. We help our patients and families to celebrate a life even as death approaches. Today, as every day, we host and we serve at the feast before the famine.

Inviting the Grim Reaper

I was helping some friends plan their wedding the other day. When we got to the vows, the bride-to-be said that she wanted the traditional vows, but would prefer to leave out the "'til death do us part language." Not because she doesn't expect the marriage to last the rest of their lives, but because she didn't want to mention death at the wedding, didn't want to put the grim reaper on the invite list.

Though happy to accommodate her request, I couldn't help but tell her that she may not want death at her wedding, but death is an awful party guest. It shows up even when it isn't invited; it takes attention away from the bride, mixes tears in among the laughter. Death, like any bad wedding guest, tries to make everything at the event about itself. But for all the efforts to keep death out, at every wedding, as in every other major life event, death shows up.

Death shows up in a mother's eyes whose deepest wish is that Dad could have been there to see their kid all grown up. Death show up in Grandpa's heart, who knew just how much his wife wanted to dance on that day. Death is there in the empty seat next to Uncle Joe, and in the salty tears Aunt Ruth is dabbing off her cheek. Death is there in a grandma stooped by age and approaching the end of her time on this earth, and death is there in face of a new child, whose very features carry within them the imprint of generations gone by.

The fact of the matter is that death is there at every wedding, every baptism, every graduation, every bar mitzvah, and even every birth. At important times death will not be left out, and its presence will bring up memories to all those gathered. Some of these memories will be of a loved one's last day, and each of you will be part of some of those memories. While the recollections may be painful, they do not have to be of pain.

These memories of the deceased's last day on this earth could be of struggle or slumber, of lives torn from this earth in anguish or peacefully surrendered in comfort, of last days spent loving and being loved or hurting and being tormented. You give the wedding gift of peace. Your contribution to the celebration is the eternal memory that the loved one left this earth well cared for and comforted. That Is a gift that can appear on no registry, that does not come wrapped up in a bow, and yet is more important and far greater than anything anyone could ask for.

Scarred Beauty

Unbroken things can be pretty but are never beautiful. The clean and unblemished can capture the eye, but it cannot stir the heart or move another to tears.

During Sunday service, members of my church volunteer to sing verses of the Psalm for the day. There are a few good singers in the church, but none of them volunteer. Each singing voice cries out off-key—some are raspy, others stumble over words, each voice filled with the pain and joy that make up the singer's life. It doesn't sound good; the song isn't pretty, but it's beautiful.

My dog stinks, no matter how much you bathe him, or how long you brush his teeth—he stinks. His coat doesn't shine. He is a mix of who knows how many breeds. His tail is too long, his legs too short, his snout grey, his eyes watery. He would win no dog show. Otis is an ugly mutt, but what he lacks in breeding he makes up for in sweetness and gentleness. Otis may not be pretty, but he's beautiful.

The things of this world that impact us, the things which we chose not to forget but make permanent space for in our minds, are rarely perfect. They are moments of struggle and loss, they are people who were challenges, times that have hurt. That which we hold on to and find meaning in is that which touches our soul. It is not the simple pretty things of the world, but instead the broken beauties that move our spirits.

In being with the dying we are privy to this sacred beauty. Deathbeds and hospital rooms contain scenes of beauty Picasso could not have painted, beauty found in the love between the dying and the living. Found in the care given, in the stories shared, in the struggle faced together. Death may not be pretty, but should we only look, we may stumble upon the endless and broken beauty born anew at the end of life.

Best Laid Plans

Lou was a hard worker, like many immigrants to this country; through tireless effort and constant struggle he built a business and with his wife, Ann, raised their son. There were sacrifices, long hours, sore muscles, and worried families, but Lou and his wife Ann had lived their lives well. As retirement approached, Lou and Ann made plans. Lou was nearing 70, but a lifetime of work had kept his body strong and spry. Ann was 15 years his junior and could more than keep up. They would travel to the old world and spend time in northern Italy where Lou grew up; they would ski the Alps, eat in Parisian restaurants, sip coffee in the shadow of the Acropolis. They planned to see it all, but as the expression goes, we make plans and God laughs.

Ann was diagnosed with a degenerative brain disease and, slowly, the once vivacious woman was trapped within the confines of her frame, losing even her ability to communicate. Ann was placed on hospice service in 2009 and died in 2012, Lou never away from her side. Sure, he could have traveled—they had a 24-hour caregiver and their son to look after Ann, but how could Lou go? The Eiffel tower would just be twisted metal without her standing below it, the Coliseum a pile of worthless rock fit to be tossed aside to make room for new condo construction. The Sistine Chapel would just be some pictures on a ceiling, St Peter's Basilica just a dome without her to share them with.

So they stayed in their little bungalow, which was modest enough, but to Lou, having Ann there made it more important than any great and storied palace in Europe. They may not have been able to live out their plans, but Ann and Lou did get to live together until the end. It makes you wonder why we make plans at all. Why, when the only certain thing about the future is that it will not be what we expect it to be—that interruptions from promotions at work to sudden death will change our course in life over and over again. I don't know why we make plans, but I know the same motivation that leads us to plan for a beautiful future with the ones we love is the same motivation that gives us the strength to struggle through a painful death together. That motivation is love. And that makes God smile.

Hands

Emily was a hard case. One of the growing number of the institutionalized, the orphans of the nursing home, the forgotten people. Whatever family she had had long since disappeared, her friends unwilling or unable to care for her. Though only thirty-six when I met her, her illness had already robbed her of her speech and her strength. Emily had been left in the mercy of strangers' hands with no way to stand up for herself, and at least some of those strangers did not prove merciful. The first time the nurse reached out to change a dressing, Emily, who seemed incapable of even the slightest movement, shuffled away from her hands in primal fear. For Emily, whose plight is all too common and whose abuse is all too normal, those strangers' hands had become weapons, and touch had become violence.

A tool on its own is neither good nor bad; it is only potential. A hammer could build a hospital or crack a skull, a scalpel could be used to heal or kill, a pen could write a love letter or sign a declaration of war. The tool in and of itself is nothing more than an artifact; what matters is how we use it.

Such is the case with the greatest tools we have been given—our hands. After Emily came, service hands began to take on a new meaning to her. Through the loving and kind care of hospice nurses and aids, touches were no longer painful, but soothing, their presence slowly invoking more comfort than fear, the violence Emily had experienced slipped through loving fingers. By the time she died, Emily welcomed the touch, and there she found final comfort.

I hope that Emily's case in this world is rare, though I fear it isn't. May it stand as an example of who you are and what your hands can do. Continue to choose to use your hands for healing and continue to make your touch that of comfort. Today, as you reach out for the flesh of another, pause and remind yourself that this touch may be their last. May they find comfort in your hands.

Lake Itasca

Should you ever make your way up the Mississippi, should you buck the current of the American River Ganges and play a Johnny Cash song in reverse, where the water ends you will find a line of stones rubbed smooth by the subtle but endless trickle of water from Lake Itasca. Just one lake of 10,000, a little larger than most, but nothing special on its own. Lake Itasca is the source, the mother of the great water course, home to the true headwaters of the Mississippi River. This line of smoothed stones marks the border between the still world of the lake and the beautifully chaotic flow of the river.

Our patients are like the lake, fluid and changing but always confined within the borders of themselves, the unity of solid flesh confining a single spirit. The river is shades of death; it holds the flow from broken borders where all things merge into one, a thousand lakes bleeding together, order transfigured into chaos. In the river the stillness of the many becomes the flow of the one.

We who care for the dying are that line of rocks made smooth by the water's trickle. We are that which eases the transition between the lake and the river, between this world and the next. We help to ease the pain or borders breaking, of the order a person has known becoming the chaos of that which lies beyond knowledge. It is a sacred and holy task to help one gently flow from life into death.

The Broken Plane

I sat down with an old man the other day and he spoke about his life. His beginnings in a rural town were glossed over with words like "good" and "average." When he got to his brother's death, he paused and the tears welled up. He went on to describe how he left home and joined the service. The years were covered in a few quick sentences spoken without much feeling, but then a pause again as he described his first date with his wife, and that he told in perfect detail, a mischievous grin spread across his wrinkled face. From then the story continued, years told in seconds and short moments dragged out for hours. Moments like the birth of his children and grandchildren. The death of a child, times of deep pride and love, and instances of deep regret and loss. His story fell into a rhythm where years were told in a word and mere moments were given thick, rich detail. It all finally culminated in the painful story of his wife's death.

A life is not a progression; it is not a building up over the years, nor is it a narrative of rising and falling action. Life is a line broken, a perfectly flat pain marked and scarred here and there by solitary mountains and deep ravines. These are the good or bad—the moments we dwell on. The moments that have meaning and do not fall back into the minutia of daily life, these are the places that break the plane, that interrupt the normal. Here is meaning; these powerful seconds are what make up a life. True life is not found in the things that work every time, but meaningful life is found in the broken places, the heights and the pits of our time on this earth.

So is the case with a death. We may strive for a perfect progress, to guide our patients through a predictable and controlled process, but we know there is no perfection in death. There is no unbroken line. Each and every death charts is own course, despite our best efforts. In talking with the bereaved, one thing remains in their minds above all else: our care in the crisis, our attention in the interruptions. It is in these darkest places that your lights have shone most bright. It is in the broken and cracked that the grieving have known your care. It is a great falsehood to strive for perfection, the unattainable unbroken line. Perfection is chasing the wind, an empty task and a fool's earned. What we need much more than the perfect is a light in the darkness, a companion with us on the heights and in the pits. That is who you are.

Never Alone

I spent last Wednesday night in the hospital. I was sick, scared, tired, lost, in pain and confused, and it wasn't me in the hospital bed, it was my boy. A stomach illness had made him dehydrated and infection had clogged his ears. It really wasn't all that bad, but the doc thought a night in the hospital, a bag or two of fluids and some antibiotics were the cure for what ailed him. So there we were, the two of us, him in a gown, me in sweats, him with a needle in his arm to give him fluids, me with a wound in my soul from watching them put that needle in.

When night fell and we were left alone with only the blinking lights, faint cries of other patients, and the endless beeping of the IV to keep us company, it became obvious who the real patient was. Though Hugh had cried when they placed the IV and hollered when they drew his blood, he had since drifted off into a heavy slumber. I was left awake, paging the nurse every hour or so, claiming my son had "rolled over on the call light, but as long as she was there." I was nervous and scared. I had questions and concerns, some legit, but most the panicked thoughts of an uninformed and ill-equipped man.

There is never one patient—we are never ill alone. When one of us is sick we are all infected. When one of us dies we all lose a piece of ourselves. In caring for the dying you allow yourself to become infected, you give up that piece of yourself, you feel another's pain, you take a part of another's struggle and in doing so make that struggle a little easier. This giving of yourself for the other should not be overlooked. It is not easy to join another in illness and in death, but it is a calling, and through each of you it can be the greatest of blessings.

Clearing a Path

I woke up to snow on Sunday morning. A thick coating of thin flecks of ice that nature, in its indifferent might, had decided to place in our way. A new task given, a new problem to manage, a new obstacle to remove. So I shoveled, and of course, as soon as I finished, the snow had been replaced, the driveway and sidewalk white again with fresh powder. The effort put in was hidden from sight, the perfectly cleaned and cleared concrete covered and buried by undifferentiated white.

So the day went on and the Sisyphean task of shoveling continued. Muscle versus nature, will versus law. Nature continued to win. After hours of this, my body hurt; I was cold and wet, tired and annoyed, just like everyone in a blizzard. As I prepared to go out for a fifth time, as I looked at the new fallen snow piled high once again on the sidewalk, my heart sank and my back screamed. Then I heard from outside the faint rumble of a motor, and I saw through the curtain of snow my neighbor pushing his snow blower along my stretch of sidewalk. The job wasn't perfect, and by the time he had finished his pass, the snow was already filling the path back in, but it gave me a reprieve, let me rest, and made me stronger for the task ahead. It was a small act of another that made a huge difference to me.

When our patients are diagnosed, when they are given only months to live, it is like waking up in a blizzard—burden and pain lay thick all around, having appeared from the ether. Those burdens continue to pile up. Beyond the fear and pain that go along with approaching death comes the financial concerns, caregiving issues, physical and emotional limitations, normal human fatigue and weakness. We help ease those burdens. We cannot make it perfect—no death can be—perfection is spitting into the wind, is pushing the boulder, but we can offer reprieve. We can clear a path, make a pass, and in doing so we can strengthen them for the task ahead and make a crushing load bearable—and that is no small thing.

Brackish Water

This year we spent Thanksgiving in Florida, where my old man has retired. Florida for the holidays leaves much to be desired—palms make poor Christmas trees—but every time I visit that strange southern state there is a fascination with and a draw to the mangroves. Those squat jungles, those floating forests that thrive in the brackish waters, half salt and half fresh, just on the edge of the tamed and living land and the endless wilderness of the ocean beyond.

In some of the most ancient mythology there existed two proto-gods, two things from which our reality and everything in it found its genesis. One was fresh water, representing life, the other salt water, the harbinger of death. The brackish water, the place where the life of fresh water meets the non-life of the salt, there is the place of transition, the stage in which life and death occurs. Florida is full of brackish water and life is scarce where it is found, except for the mangroves, which make this place between life and death their home. Not tall, but wide and sturdy, spread out in green jungles both firmly rooted and floating on the sea. Where life comes to die the mangrove can grow, and like that most famous of mustard seeds, it branches can become home to the birds of the air, and it roots safety to the fish of the sea. The mangrove makes room for life even in the face of death. The mangrove is the hospice of the natural world.

As the mangrove is to the birds and fish, so may we be for our patients and their families. May our hands be branches of safety and shelter. May our skill be a shade of love offering comfort from the elements. May our presence provide shelter in a frightening time. May we be rooted in the knowledge that our care is powerful and meaningful. My we stand as a firm foundation for those traversing the waters of life and the waters of death.

Strength

It was my job to help out Tommy. Six-foot-two and 150 pounds soaking wet with his clothes on. Tommy was 21, give or take five years. I was working with a group providing meals and support to the homeless on the street, and Tommy was amongst their ranks. He was nothing but sinew, bone and blonde hair, all of which was stumbling and belligerent. Drunk or worse, Tommy was a real piece of work, cursing and shouting on a public street, scaring people and causing trouble. It may have been the booze or the drugs talking, but I wanted them to shut up. Just as I was about to make this point clear in the most unhelpful of ways, Joe stepped in.

An older man, himself homeless, dirty, and ragged by polite society standards, Joe wrapped a ropey arm around Tommy and led him away. A few minutes later I saw the two in the park. Tommy was sitting up and talking, and Joe was patiently listening. The angry mess of booze and trouble had become a calm, though still confused young man talking with a kind and helpful elder in Joe. Here I was, a professional nice guy with the clinical residencies and silly letters behind my name to prove how good I was, and this old homeless man in a matter of seconds was able to care for someone I could not even talk to.

There is strength in others we do not give them credit for. There are powers buried deep down in the basements of our very souls that can do things we, in our calmer moments, could not dream of. Our patients' families are made up of people who, for the most part, have never seen a person die, let alone cared for the dying. I would wager if you were to ask them outside of the situation if they could do such an act, most would say no. Our families more often than not are able to dig deep into their souls and pull out of their storehouses the strength and love to care for their dying. We help them to find that strength; we guide them to those places of love and care and support tucked away inside of them. May we always have confidence that our families have the strength to care for others, because each person is powerful, we just need to help them find where to look.

Interruptions

On Saturdays, if the weather is palatable, we make our way down to 114th street just west of Archer Ave. Millions of years ago a retreating glacier left a huge pile of stones, creating an elevated ridge in our otherwise flat Midwestern plane. Today that ridge is part of the Cook County forest preserve. A toboggan run was built into the hill nearly a century ago. To access the top of the run, an uneven set of limestone steps were carved into the ridge.

The toboggan run has long since been shut down, but these steps remain, a staircase to nothing that draws thousands to this strange spot. People come from all over; every creed and color can be found climbing those hundreds of steps. Sweating on their way up and panting on their way down, over and over again. A bit of exercise and a chance to be out in nature brings us all together. After a few times up the steps, between gulps of air and drops of sweat, you can't help but notice the metaphor in it all. The stairs as life. No matter who we are or where we come from, we are bound to the repetitive nature of existence. The joy in achieving a goal, the pain in the struggle to reach the top, the disappointment in not getting as far as you want. All of this is seen in miniature as the people work their way up and down the staircase. Like Sisyphus with his boulder, each of us get up day after day, set to the rhythm of climbing and descending the stairs to nowhere that are our lives.

This rhythm of up and down is always in danger of interruption. Every so often someone on the stairs will push themselves a little too hard and need to stop halfway up, or a person will trip descending the jagged stones. These are usually minor incidents, but every interruption carries danger; one sudden stop or one stumble down the stairs can start a chain reaction. One person's misstep can send them colliding with another, bringing on a domino effect causing all to tumble. The thing about an abandoned staircase in the middle of nowhere is that when everyone starts to fall, there is no one around to stop it.

Just as the rhythm of the steps is a metaphor for life, so the interruption, the falling down, is a metaphor for death. In death an outside event, a loss of a loved one, can send lives careening out of control. The loss of one person can cause entire groups of people to fall into chaos. The difference is on the steps there is no one to soften the landing. In our care we can cushion the fall. When their lives start to tumble out of control, we may not be able to stop the motion, but we can grab on to them, hold them close and ease them to the ground. In doing so we can keep catastrophe at bay and set the stage for a new rhythm in their life to begin.